FROM
FEAR
TO
FAITH

Surviving

Cancer

Six

Times

RUTH ORR

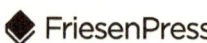 FriesenPress

One Printers Way
Altona, MB R0G 0B0
Canada

www.friesenpress.com

Scripture quotations are taken from the Holy Bible, New Living Translation, copyright 1996,2004,2007,2013 by Tyndale House Foundation. Used by permission of Tyndale House Publishers, Inc., Carol Stream, Illinois 60188.

Poem- Burden's Lifted by Edith Clattenburg. Unpublished. Used by permission.

ISBN
978-1-03-915695-1 (Hardcover)
978-1-03-915694-4 (Paperback)
978-1-03-915696-8 (eBook)

1. BIOGRAPHY & AUTOBIOGRAPHY, PERSONAL MEMOIRS

Distributed to the trade by The Ingram Book Company

DEDICATION

THIS BOOK IS DEDICATED TO ALL
THOSE WHO HAVE HEARD THE WORDS
"You have cancer".

May the fear that grips you, become the
faith that sustains you.

Cancer. That dreaded word. It invokes fear every time we hear it. And we hear it almost daily. Eat this and you won't get cancer; don't eat this, it causes cancer. We live in a constant state of fear, and it motivates us to make decisions and choices out of fear.

When you hear the words "You have cancer," you cross over the fence and join all those who have heard those words spoken to them. Life takes on a different perspective from that side. For those who have crossed over that fence, life is not the same. It's often referred to as BC and AC—Before Cancer and After Cancer. Your focus now on how to deal with it.

I have heard those words six times in my life. In the span of three years, I had five surgeries. I know about the world of cancer. I know about surgeries, radiation, chemotherapy, CAT scans, PET scans, horrible-tasting drinks, IVs, and blood counts. I know the blue gown goes on first and ties in the back, and the green one goes over it and ties in the front, and it's important to get it right. I know what it is like to sit in a waiting room full of other people dressed in the same gowns, all pretending we're not naked underneath. I know what it's like to say goodbye to your hair and to see the first visible signs that you have cancer. I know what it's like to look in the faces of loved ones and realize their fear is bigger than mine. Most importantly, I have learned to face fear. I could not control what was happening to me, but I could choose how I responded.

FROM FEAR TO FAITH.
This is my journey.

CHAPTER 1
THE JOURNEY BEGINS

December 24, 2004. My feet hit the floor, and I was getting ready to face the day. Already my head was working out the details and schedule for the day. It was Christmas Eve, and there were lots of preparations yet to make. Cleaning, wrapping, baking, and all the last-minute things. As I was getting dressed, the phone rang. It was my doctor calling.

That moment seems to be suspended in time. He had just gotten the biopsy report back that morning and had to call to let me know they had found cancer cells in the breast tissue they had tested. He went on to tell me all kinds of other stuff after that, and then he paused. "Have I lost you?" he asked.

"Yes," I replied, "back there when you said they found cancer." My mind was stuck. Frozen on those words in that moment. It had been an anxious time leading up to this day. I had been recalled for a second mammogram, ultrasound, and a biopsy that was done in the weeks prior and, of course, I had been hoping the reports would be negative—especially when it had been almost two weeks since I had heard anything. And no news is good news, or so I thought.

In my frozen state of shock, my brain tried to process this information. Numbly, I continued to do the tasks that I had been doing before the call. I dressed, did my hair, and got ready for the day. Then I proceeded downstairs to face my husband who was waiting to hear the news.

It hit me when I told him because the words were coming out of my mouth. I then melted into his arms and the tears came like a flood. I was so scared.

After the initial shock, my brain kicked in and reminded me that regardless of the news, Christmas was still coming and there were things to do. So, I went about doing them, trying to keep my focus on the tasks at hand.

I have come to realize that the worst place to be is when you are first diagnosed. At that time, all I knew is that I had unwanted cells in my body, and I wanted them out—NOW! Unfortunately, I had to wait to meet with the doctor and find out the plan of action. Waiting is always the hardest.

My most favourite time of Christmas is Christmas Eve, when everything is done, and the celebration begins. First, it's church. The best way to begin Christmas is celebrating the one who is the person of honour—Jesus. My faith has always been my strength and source throughout my life, and I knew I needed that faith now more than ever to see me through.

That evening was tough though. I did not want to tell everyone and ruin their Christmas. But I did tell a few close friends as I knew they would be praying for me. My pastor spoke to me about being a warrior and said that I would fight this battle and show everyone how to walk through this with faith. I remember thinking, *I do not feel like a warrior. I feel weak and scared and helpless.*

As I think back on this, I realize that a warrior goes into battle not courageously, but weak and scared and helpless, and they find a strength within that is God-given.

The holiday season passed, and I somehow managed to get through it. The fear was still overwhelming, and I did a lot of praying. I knew that God would: A, deliver me from; or B, see me through it. I chose plan A, and God chose plan B.

At the beginning of the new year, I met with my surgeon. My fear was lessened some as now I was given a plan of action. I would have a lumpectomy, followed by radiation.

The surgery took place a few weeks later. What a feeling of relief when I knew the cancer had been taken out.

A week later, I went back to get the report. It was good news. All the cancer had been removed, and there was none in the lymph nodes. However, because it was an aggressive tumour and I was a young woman, the doctor recommended that I have chemotherapy as well as radiation. She was concerned about the long term.

That word, CHEMOTHERAPY! It was bigger than the word cancer and not just in the number of letters. It brought a whole new wave of fear to me. My immediate thought went to my daughter's wedding, which was to take place that summer. I was now going to have treatments with a drug that would make me sick and cause me to lose my hair, and I would probably die. You see, that was my grid for chemo. That was all I had ever seen. My doctor, however, saw a different picture. She saw people all the time who have had treatments and survived and even thrived after. When I mentioned the wedding to her, she just casually replied, "You can wear a wig; you will be fine."

I have to say that at this point, I was not ready for this news. Having surgery and radiation, although uncomfortable, were not visual to the world. The side effects were minimal. But chemotherapy was a whole different ballgame. As a woman, losing my hair was a huge deal. Not so much as a pride issue, but it was a visual sign that announced to the world that I had cancer. I had always had a tremendous respect for doctors and health care professionals, but at that moment, I came close to hitting a doctor. I numbly left the hospital with my husband and sister-in-law, and I cried all the way home.

For the next few weeks, while waiting to meet with an oncologist, I spent time reading my Bible, which was a real source of comfort for me. Even though I did not understand why I was having to walk through this illness and why God did not heal me, I found comfort in reading about people of faith who were not without their struggles. As I found solace in my reading, there were certain passages that I began to read over and over.

- "I will never leave you or forsake you." (Hebrews 13:5)
- "Even though I walk through death's dark valley, I will be with you to comfort you." (Psalm 23:4)
- "Because you have made the Lord your God, your dwelling place, no evil will come near you. He will give his angels charge over you to keep you in all your ways." (Psalm 91:9-11)
- "I would have lost heart, had I not believed, I would see the goodness of God in the land of the living." (Psalm 27:13)

I started to keep a journal at this point—not just of my thoughts and feelings, but of the things I was grateful for. There is power in being thankful no matter the circumstances. It changes your attitude and realigns your focus to what is good, not the bad stuff. Remember the image of the little angel on one shoulder whispering good things in your ear while the devil is on the other whispering bad things? What you believe is what you listen to and give attention to. It was time for me to knock that little devil off my shoulder and not listen to him. If God said He would see me through, He would.

I met with my oncologist a few weeks later and got the plan of action. Oncologists are a special breed of doctor. They take the time to explain everything and listen to your concerns. I left his office feeling that I could do this and get through it. There was a plan now, and I knew what to expect.

I was to have four chemo treatments, each with three weeks between them. The side effects were nausea and vomiting for forty-eight hours, but with the help of good anti-nausea drugs, I would get through. There would be a ninety-five percent hair loss, and they can tell you to the day when it will start to fall out. My immune system would be weakened, so I was told to stay out of crowds where people are sick. Those were the biggies. Knowing what you must do to survive puts you in a mind-set to get this train going and get it over with.

One thing was bothering me though. I HATE needles! I can't even watch them being put into someone else. When they show this simple procedure on TV, I turn my head. I had thought about being a nurse when I was young, but the needle issue was a dealbreaker. There was no way I was going to be able to stick a needle in someone and have them pick me up off the floor. The chemo nurses have a special *touch*, and they would do their best to alleviate my fears.

I remember that first treatment well. As I watched that red drug, which looked like a bag of Kool-Aid going in my veins, I wondered if I would glow in the dark that night. (Of course, I checked that out—I didn't.) I did not want to know the toxic chemicals that were in it, only that it would do the job and kill the bad cells. I was in a room with only one other person, and she was not doing well, so I decided to be selective in whom I talked to. I had friends who became my chemo buddies, and they would keep me on a positive vibe. I got sick only once after that first treatment and was able to function well after twenty-four hours. I decided to arm myself with hand sanitizer and go shopping. I realized that life was not going to stop because I had cancer, so I had to learn to function with it. I could not change what was happening to me, but I could adjust my attitude on how I responded. That is where I found my power.

My motto each morning was get up, get dressed, get cute, and get out. Being involved in the beauty industry for years and as a business woman, I knew that when you look good you feel better. So, I made sure I looked my best, not for anyone else, but for me. I knew I could control this important aspect of my life. My hairdresser and friend asked me if I wanted help in choosing a wig, and I said, "yes." So, off we went to purchase a wig. What fun we had that day. I have pictures of many different styles; we laughed at so many of them and finally settled for one that was not too far off from my normal hairdo. I was ready for that inevitable day when my hair would fall out.

Those unmistakable wisps of hair on the pillow told me it was time. Even though you know it's coming, a part of you says maybe, just maybe, I will be spared. I will be the one in a million who does not lose my hair. But there it was on the pillow. Like Dorothy in the Wizard of Oz, I saw the writing in the sky, "surrender Ruth," let go of that hair. When it was falling out, my scalp was tender, so I did what was recommended and had it buzzed off. My hairdresser took me privately and did the job. There are no words to describe how you feel when you look in the mirror and see where your hair used to be. Many times, I passed by a mirror and asked myself, "who is this person?"

The wig was fitted and placed on my head. *Not bad*, was my first thought as I looked in the mirror. But did it look real?

Would people immediately see that it was a wig? Would it blow off with a gust of wind? I had a whole different set of fears now. I found out that the tabs on the sides of the wig, which you use to make sure it's straight, are great to hold on to when it gets windy. I just pretended I was covering my ears.

I had a lot of fun with my wig. There are advantages to wearing one. Fixing the back of my hair was a whole lot easier when I could just take the wig off and flip it around. I saved a lot of money on haircuts. My wig kept my head warm when it was cold, and when it got hot, I took it off. I loved the reactions of people when I did this—especially when I said something like "I'd forget my head if it wasn't glued on."

My wig was made of a synthetic material, which meant I could not wear it in the kitchen while I was cooking, or it would frizzle and melt. So, I always removed it and set it on the back of the big armchair in the living room. My daughter would think I was sitting in the chair and have a conversation with me until she realized I was not there but in the kitchen. The dog was suspicious of it though, and he would bark at it. The cat would have taken it away if she'd had the chance. Whenever we were getting ready to go out somewhere, my daughters would be searching for their hairbrushes, and I would be searching for my hair. Wearing a wig and makeup when I went out gave me some control. I got to choose how I looked and who I wanted to talk to about my ordeal.

The chemo cycle became routine. Every three weeks, I went into the hospital for the treatment. The next forty-eight hours I would take the anti-nausea drugs. I felt crappy for twenty-four hours and then tried to function as normally as possible. I ate whatever I could, whenever I could. I kept sick people at a distance and used lots of hand sanitizer. I managed to finish my treatments on schedule and then moved on to the next part, which was radiation.

Radiation. After chemo, radiation is supposed to be a walk in the park, or so they say. It is just different. I had twenty-five treatments, one every day for five days a week. Because I lived about forty kilometres from the hospital, it meant I had to travel into the city each day, find a parking space, change into one of those famous hospital gowns, and wait for my turn on the big machine. It took about ten minutes to get me into position and ninety seconds for the actual treatment. It was fine at first, but after about number sixteen, I started to feel the burn. By the time number twenty-five came, I was a crispy critter. My final treatment was on July the 8th. My daughter's wedding was on July 16th. It certainly was a great celebration.

One of the things I was told was that my energy level would be low and I would need lots of rest. I was not sure what that would look like for me with my family. My husband, Dave, was a long-distance truck driver; Melanie was a college student and the bride; and Rebecca was graduating high school. There were proms, showers, graduations, parties, and family gatherings. My prayer (after "this can't be happening to me at this time") was that God would give me the strength to not just endure, but enjoy all the events. I was present for all the festivities and enjoyed every moment. I learned that walking through tough stuff made me stronger. I felt like the warrior after the battle was done, and I was victorious. Oh yes, at the wedding I danced until midnight, kicked off my shoes, and hung my hair on the chair!

CHAPTER 2

Fast-forward ten years. Dave and I went on our dream vacation to Hawaii and then returned there in 2013 with friends. We had a wonderful time exploring the islands from excursions on the cruise ship. Both of our daughters were now married. We had two wonderful grandchildren and another on the way. I felt truly blessed. Life was good and I was enjoying it to the fullest. I had no idea grandchildren could bring so much joy. It's like parenting without the responsibility. My children informed me that their children were not allowed ice cream before supper. I guess I forgot the rules.

In October of 2014, I turned that magical age of sixty. OK, maybe not magical. Dave and I took a little road trip around Nova Scotia. I was not feeling well but thought I had just eaten something that disagreed with me. Upon returning home, I started bleeding from the bowel. Not wanting to go to emergency, I went to a walk-in clinic and was told to go to the ER right away. Of course, it was nighttime and the wait was long. When I did get in, the bleeding had stopped, and I figured they would send me home. Nope, that was not the case.

I was admitted that night and prepped for a colonoscopy the next day, which they did not have time to do, so I had to wait in hospital over the weekend until they could do the test on Monday. This delay meant that I had to go through the prep work again on Sunday. I was all cleaned out and a few pounds lighter. What they did not tell me was that they had done the blood work to check the cancer tumour levels in my body, which can indicate if there is colon cancer present. The normal level is two, mine was ten.

I remember this young intern coming into my room and sitting on the bed while he told me I had a large, suspicious tumour on my colon. They were pretty sure it was cancerous. I looked at the intern's face and saw the fear in his eyes. I realized this could be the first time he had ever been given the task of telling a patient bad news. I felt sorry for him. I looked him in the eye and touched his hand and said that God and I had done this battle before, and we would do it again. The relief on his face was evident; he was glad that I had a positive attitude about it.

However, that was not how I was feeling inside. The swirl of emotions circled around in me, and again I was faced with that fear. My mind was reliving the previous experience with cancer and wondering if I could go through that again. I was also looking ahead and hoping to see my grandchildren grow up. Telling my family was hard—seeing the fear on their faces and realizing there was nothing I could do to calm them.

I started to read the old scriptures I had read during the last battle, but I did not feel any comfort. This was a different battle, and I needed a new battle plan to help me fight. I knew the doctors and oncologists would have a plan of action for the physical needs. I needed to take care of my mental and spiritual needs. Doctors can tell you all about the side effects of treatments, but only the one who walks through the ordeal can tell you the psychological side effects.

I started to look at other passages of scripture for strength and healing. I read until I found the ones I needed this time— the ones that would grip my heart as I read them. Two stood out for me. The first one was Isaiah 41:10: "Do not be afraid, for I am with you. Do not be discouraged, for I am your God. I will strengthen you and help you. I will hold you up with my victorious right hand." The second one was Psalm 40:1-3: "I waited patiently for the Lord to help me, and he turned to me and heard my cry. He lifted me out of the pit of despair, out of the mud and the mire. He set my feet on solid ground and steadied me as I walked along. He has given me a new song to sing, a hymn of praise to our God. Many will see what he has done and be amazed. They will put their trust in the Lord."

My part was to not be afraid, not be discouraged, and to wait patiently. God's part was that He would be with me. He would strengthen and help me and hold me up, lift me out of the pit, set my feet on solid ground, and steady me as I walked. In my first battle with cancer, I was the warrior. This time God was telling me this battle was His. Somehow, I knew I was going to make it through. My mind was prepared before the doctors knew what they were dealing with.

My surgeon decided to do a CT scan, which was followed by a PET scan. One tells if there are any other spots in the body, and the other tells if they are cancerous. Bad news. It had already spread to my liver. I had stage four colon cancer. I now had two surgeons who were planning a double surgery.

I remember asking God how deep this pit was going to get and then remembering the scripture that He would lift me out of the pit. I realized there was no pit too deep for God to get me out of.

The surgery was five hours, and I spent eleven days in hospital. They removed two tumours. During my stay in hospital,

I was put in a room with three other patients, and for most of the stay they were male. We had one washroom. You can hear if someone washes their hands after using the bathroom, and no offence guys, but you're not the best at doing that. As I lay there, I knew that when I needed to go, I had to clean before using.

I was released from hospital on December 15, 2014, and my granddaughter Elizabeth was born on the 18th. What a joy it was to be able to focus on someone else and not on my problems. The moment I held her was such a special time.

As Christmas approached, I spent my time resting and recuperating as I could not do much. Watching others in my kitchen preparing Christmas dinner was a unique experience. It had always been me rushing around doing the preparations. Sometimes letting go can be a good thing. The table was full with lots of food and family around. I was filled with joy and thanksgiving.

When trials come my way, they never seem to come one at a time. There are always a few together. My daughter Rebecca and her husband, Nick, and two grandchildren were planning to move. Nick is in the military, and they were moving to Yellowknife in the Northwest Territories—about six thousand kilometres away! Needless to say, it was a very difficult time for me. I was not sure what the treatment plan was going to be and did not know what my survival chances were, so it was hard to watch them prepare to go. I knew it would be exciting for them and they had family for support there, but I could not share in their joy of adventure in this endeavour. Having loved ones around you is so important to help in the healing process. My heart ached.

For anyone who lived in Eastern Canada, we remember the winter of 2015. It was absolute snowmageddon! We had close to five-hundred centimetres of snow. That is about sixteen feet. I did not see the road in front of my house for three months. The driveway was like a tunnel through the snow. You could make snow angels standing up! We averaged two storms a week.

What was happening in the natural world felt like what I was experiencing in my spiritual journey. I was overwhelmed with all that was going on. The physical healing was taking longer. Knowing that I was going to have chemotherapy again and that the kids were moving weighed heavily on me. When my physical body is not strong, it affects my spiritual life as well. Many nights when I was tired, I would sit on the side of my bed and cry. My God, who is ever present with me, would hear the cries of my heart. Then I would put my head on the pillow and sleep. That was what the peace of God looked like to me during that time. Over and over, in the book of Psalms, there are many laments of the heart, and I related to them. I realize that, in life, we would like to skip over the pain, both physical and emotional, but facing it with no understanding and crying out to God is humbling because you realize your weakness. But then you see God in His strength. I reminded myself daily that God was in control. I was to not be afraid, to not be disappointed, and to wait patiently.

My body was getting stronger as I rested and recovered. Chemotherapy started in February. This time I did not have to go to the hospital to have treatments. Instead, treatment was pills that could be taken orally at home. NO MORE NEEDLES! This treatment was much easier to handle. I experienced no hair loss, and even though there were about ten pages of side effects, my biggest problem was heartburn. That was manageable. I was so grateful for the advances in medicine, but my eyes were opened to the cost of all these drugs! Thank goodness for drug plans.

I realized that when there was nothing I could do to change the situation, I had to change how I looked at the situation. Perspective gives you focus. As I said goodbye to my family, I was already making plans to go visit.

Winter was long; spring was short; summer arrived, and finally the snow was gone. It was amazing how fast it disappeared when the warm weather hit. I thought I would be making snowballs in July.

After the treatments were all finished, I hoped things would return to normal. Your body tells you that, but your mind must adjust. When going through cancer, you go into survival mode. You do whatever it takes to survive. Your brain is in neutral. Afterwards, your brain must catch up and process what you have just gone through. This does not happen overnight. I needed time to reflect, to get direction, and to gain perspective on my life.

I let go of doing things that did not bring me joy. Well, almost everything. Dishes, meals, and the other mundane housework was still there to do, but what I could let go of, I did. The things that gave me purpose like family, my business, teaching the Bible to children and adults, and enjoying people were front and centre in my daily activities. Everyday became a special day. If a friend was coming over, I would get out the china teapot and cups and use them.

I also became more aware of what I could control and what I couldn't—what was mine to do and what was God's. Remember the Scripture verses? My part was to not be afraid, to not be discouraged, and to wait patiently. His job was to rescue me from the pit, set my feet on solid ground, and steady me as I walked. I had to learn what that looked like each day.

Dave and I went on a trip to Yellowknife that October and had a wonderful time with our children and two grandchildren.

They were just in the process of moving again. This time to Kingston, Ontario, which was a lot closer to us. You've got to love the military life. As they say, "there is no life like it."

My oldest daughter, Melanie, her husband Roland, and their son Charlie were renovating their house to sell, so they moved in with us for ten months. What fun it was to have the house full again. I was feeling well physically and enjoying life. I was so unprepared for the next chapter.

CHAPTER 3

The next winter was not nearly like the previous one. Although it was cold, there was little snow that winter, and it was bearable. I think I would like to be like a bear and just hibernate for the winter. That idea seems to make a lot of sense to me. Spring came, and I was busy with my business and teaching Sunday School. So, there was lots to occupy my time.

Every year the time comes for those routine tests. Even though I try to remain positive and upbeat, when your body has betrayed you in the past, your trust level is not there. After having a mammogram, I got a recall for a second one and a biopsy, which confirmed I had breast cancer again. This time in the other breast. From the time of the mammogram to the further testing and to meeting with a surgeon is only a few weeks, but when it is you, it seems like forever.

My reaction to this news was different than the previous times. My thoughts and my words were along the lines of: *This can't be happening to me, not three times! Come on! Haven't I had enough?* I was angry! Especially at God. How could He let this happen to me? Looking back, I can't say that I lost faith in Him, but I was disappointed and angry, so I let Him know. I remember going for a walk in the park close to where I live and angrily marching along the path. Normally I would be praying, but not that day.

Suddenly, I stopped short and looked down at the ground. Right in front of me was a snake. It was about eight inches long and had his head lifted, and he was looking at me. As I stared him down, I shooed him off the path and continued on my way.

When I got home I sat down to read my Bible passage for that day. It was in 2 Kings 19:10-20. Basically, it says this:

> The king of Jerusalem, King Hezekiah, was sent a note from the King of Assyria, who had the city surrounded and told Hezekiah basically that Jerusalem might as well surrender because the Assyrians had conquered surrounding towns and their gods of wood and stone had not protected them, and Jerusalem was next. The King of Assyria told Hezekiah there was nothing their God could do about it. King Hezekiah took the letter and laid it on the altar and prayed to God. God delivered Jerusalem because 185,000 of the enemy's army died the next night, and they retreated.

As I was thinking about this passage I heard a voice very clearly and distinctly say, "I am the god of this world and the god of cancer, and I can take you out, and I will. There is nothing your God can or will do about it."

I was used to hearing the still small voice of God and His leading by His word, but never had I heard the voice of Satan. I clearly knew it was not God's voice, and since I had put my faith in God and listened to His voice, I knew it was not a message to be believed. I told Satan that he might have authority over cancer, but not over me. I belonged to God, and He had me in the palm of His hand, and no one could pluck me from there (John 10:27-30). I told Satan to take a hike. I then saw the image of the snake slithering away. At this point, my anger dissipated. My faith meter went from zero to ten, and I felt God say, "I got this, no worries."

After having this spiritual encounter, I felt like a fighter again. I was not going to give up or give in to the fear. While I waited for the next surgery, I kept my mind focused. I read His word and spent time with family and friends. I watched crazy, silly movies that made me laugh and ate chocolate, lots of chocolate.

I met with yet another surgeon and was totally prepared to have a full mastectomy, but she said that was much too invasive and that all she needed to do was remove the lump and do follow-up radiation. No big deal. Easy for her to say. So, for the second time in a year, I went under the knife. This time, I was out of hospital on the same day as the surgery.

The radiation treatments followed in September of that year. I had sixteen treatments over three weeks. It was much easier than ten years before, but still I had to deal with the travel and traffic. I was beginning to feel my stress levels mount higher than before.

I had never attended cancer support groups, mainly because I lived outside the city, and my Mary Kay ladies became my support group. They knew how to cheer me up and hugged me when I needed it. They also filled my freezer with food on more than one occasion. My church family was a great support to me as well, and they made sure I was taken care of. They prayed continually and checked on me regularly.

However, this time I decided to talk to a counsellor. Talking to a counsellor helped me get a few more coping skills to help me through the emotional side of things. One thing I have learned is that there is plenty of support out there, and no one needs to walk through cancer alone. The Canadian Cancer Society, volunteer services, *Look Good Feel Better* program, and online resources are all available to help cancer patients. Knowing that I had friends who I could call at any time, day or night, just to talk was comforting and reassuring.

I got busy in October and November with my business. I decided to set a personal goal to earn one of those diamond rings that Mary Kay offers, not because I wanted it particularly, but it was a goal to focus on. And I needed something positive to do to keep me busy. Little did I know how much I would need that distraction.

CHAPTER 4

January 2017. Each year starts with a promise of a new beginning, which is why we always wish everyone a Happy New Year. It starts for most people with a list of resolutions or goals for the year, usually the first one is to lose a few of the pounds you put on over the holiday. My list was no exception. Lose ten pounds. I would focus on my business plan and move forward. No excuses.

January was also the month I had a scheduled CT scan. I knew this procedure would always be a part of my routine now, but I still had that anxiety. This time the results showed a new growth on my liver, and the only way to access it was to do another liver resection. Surgery AGAIN!

My surgeon informed me that he would take care of me and do this operation, but he would be leaving the hospital soon after and would not be there for the follow-up. This was difficult as he was the one whom I had trusted, and I had liked how he looked after me. (He was also good looking.)

This time I did not feel angry or afraid. It almost felt surreal, like I couldn't believe it. However, if God had pulled me through all of what I had been through, He would not leave me now. So, I kept focused on what I had set out to do—have the surgery, get better, and move on. Sounds easy.

So not. Focusing on goals and staying positive when my health was being challenged again was not easy. Living one day at a time and not focusing ahead is not a normal way to live, but it was what I was learning to do. Each day, I did what I could for that day.

They say recouping from surgery takes six weeks. That might be the case if you're twenty, but not at sixty-three. It would be May before I started to feel normal again. Or at least what I remembered normal to be. It turns out that "normal is just a setting on your dryer," as author Patsy Clairmont says (1993). Normal just becomes different. The cancer turned out to be from the original colon cancer, so it was not new, and there was no follow-up treatment. Yea! They told me they would keep a close watch on me, so if anything showed on the scans they would be able to catch it early.

I was so glad this was over and done with. In spite of the cancer, I still managed to focus on my goal in Mary Kay and accomplished it by June 30 with a little help from my friends. In fact, in six months I had completed my list of resolutions that I had made in January—even the weight goal. However, this would be the last time I would put a weight loss goal on my resolution list, unless I also specified that no surgery would be involved.

In my checkup appointments, I had the doctor look at a mole that was growing on my leg. Not taking any chances, he referred me to a dermatologist. It took six months for the referral to go through as someone lost it. By the time I saw her, she took one look at it and had me see a specialist right away. Turns out, it was melanoma.

CHAPTER 5

I was hoping, at this point, that I was having a bad dream, and I would soon wake up and life would be lovely, but that did not happen. Dave and I were going on a trip that we had planned and paid for, and we were not sure if we could go now. This time I did not have to wait long to see a surgeon. I was in his office within a week. He took off the mole and said he would probably have to do more, but not to worry; go on vacation. He would see me when I got back.

It's so easy to tell someone not to worry, but when you have been through this four times before, these are kind of a waste of words. I learned, however, throughout this journey how to live in the moment, and if I did not have to deal with something that day, I could push it from my mind. We had a wonderful road trip to Tennessee, visiting Pidgeon Forge, Nashville, and Graceland. Then we stopped in Oklahoma to visit with Dave's sister and her husband.

When I got back, I had to face the music again—another surgery. They had to make sure there were clear margins and that the cancer was not in the lymph nodes. This doctor decided to do another PET scan on me the day before the surgery. The good news was that there was no cancer in the bloodstream or the lymphatic system, but—and there was a but—they noticed a small growth on my lung, which they had thought was scar tissue. It turned out it was not. By being proactive and having a mole removed by a doctor who checked further, I now was facing something bigger—lung cancer.

If you think I was shaking my head in disbelief, so was my doctor. I kept remembering those scriptures that had held me through these trials. I still believed that God was with me and would see me through. A new verse, John 14:27, came to me. It reads, "Peace I leave with you; my peace I give you. I do not give to you as the world gives. Do not let your heart be troubled and do not be afraid."

Its's easy to feel God's peace and not be afraid when life is good. Now I was facing cancer for the sixth time, and this time it was in my lung. Would this ever stop? I realized the enemy wanted to take me out, and I was not going to give in to the fear that would change my belief in God. So, I decided that if I had to say one thousand times a day, "I will not let my heart be troubled, and I will not be afraid," I would do it until I no longer felt the fear. Speaking the Word out loud is a powerful weapon. It builds faith and hinders the plans of the enemy.

It was now Christmastime again, and I was facing another surgery. It was scheduled for January.

CHAPTER 6

"I will trust in the Lord and not be afraid." This became my daily mantra. The more I said it, the less fearful I became. I now had to bring another surgeon up-to-speed on my medical history. His words to me were, "Wow! You're still alive!"

My options were to have surgery to completely remove the tumour with no follow-up necessary, or to have a series of radiation treatments to shrink the tumour. Because I was in good health, option one was recommended.

On January 22, 2018, I went under the knife again. For three of my surgeries, I was in the same hospital and the same operating room. You say goodbye to your loved one, then walk the hall, and go up in the elevator to the hallway of the operating rooms. You are then put on a stretcher outside the room, and you wait and wait and wait. No one talks to you or even makes eye contact with you. You listen to them talk as they get ready and scrub up, and you count the ceiling tiles. If ever there was a need for pastoral care or comfort care, that would be the place for it. Even some nice soothing music or something on the ceiling to amuse you would be great. I get that the area must have limited access and be sterile, but it sure is lonely and scary. After the wait, you are taken off the stretcher and you walk into a cold operating room. They lower the table for me, quite a bit lower for me. I measure only four feet ten inches without shoes.

The masked people are all assembled and getting ready. Next comes the anesthesiologist who is looking for a good vein to start an IV. "Just one to start," I say, "then give me the drug to put me under. After that, you can put in all the needles you want." As the IV starts and the mask goes over your face, you feel yourself drifting away. You then feel that you are drifting in and out of sleep, and you hear the unmistakable beep of the machines. There is no pain, but moving any part seems to be impossible.

I spent three days in the hospital this time. I had to practice breathing exercises every day to get my lungs back in working order. It always seemed to happen that when I was in the hospital there was a major snowstorm. It made it difficult for people to visit and lonely for me. I was glad to get home again and to start recuperating. I looked at my bruised and battered body, and all I could say was, "Well, at least I'm alive."

There are times when you feel that your body will never heal or feel better, but it does. Physical scars remain, but the body does an amazing job of healing itself. The mind is another matter.

My friends and family were always there for support, but sometimes I felt alone and that no one understood what I was going through. That's because they had not gone through it. Reaching out to someone who was experiencing cancer was risky because I was afraid to get too close in case things were not going well with them, and I did not want to think about that. When you're focused on getting better and healing, it's hard to be around someone who is not doing well. So, I did not take that chance. I am not sure I would recommend that, as support can be very powerful and helpful. But I sense that a lot of people feel the same way. If I were to give advice, I would tell people not to be afraid of reaching out for support. However, I turned to God to help me and give me strength instead.

My daughter and her family were posted back to Halifax, and I was excited to have them back. Nothing lifts my spirit up like my grandchildren. What joy they bring to my life! I now have five precious ones and love to spend time with them, although they can quickly tire me out. Where they get their energy, I do not know.

CHAPTER 7

It has been almost five years since my last surgery. This is the longest period I have gone through with no recurrences. My scans have been clear and I have been feeling great. My follow-up schedule is in place, and I feel at peace.

One thing I have learned is to listen to my body. When it is tired, I rest. I try to eat as healthily as I can. I love to eat, especially chocolate, but I am very aware of what fuel I put in. In listening to my body, I have become aware of what foods can cause my body to not function properly. So, I eliminate those foods. I also try to walk everyday or exercise on my treadmill. I make sure I cover up in the sun or wear sunscreen.

I have learned to continually check my attitude to make sure it stays positive. I read things that are uplifting and make sure I laugh every day. One positive thing that has come out of this experience is that now I never seem to have a bad hair day. I remember back to looking in the mirror when my hair was buzzed off, and now I say, "a bad hair day beats a no hair day, any day."

Most of all, I have learned to trust God more than ever in my life. I have learned that even in the hard stuff, one word of assurance can calm my frazzled nerves and give me an unexplainable peace. When I look at what is going on in the world around me and listen to the fear that people have about the future, or the climate change, the political unrest, the fighting, I see things from a different perspective. I see an unchanging God who is in control, loves me deeply, and holds me in the palm of His hand. I realize that I have been given life and life abundantly, and it is my choice on how to live that out. I choose to live it joyously and victoriously. I don't know what the future holds, but I know who holds my future. And when fear creeps in, as it will do at times, I go to my friend Jesus who is always there.

My wonderful sister-in-law, Edith, who was always helpful to me during my journey, wrote several poems for me to read while I recuperated. The one included here was special to me as it summed up my spiritual journey and how God lifted my burdens and took me from fear to faith.

BURDENS LIFTED

My burdens were heavy,
I could feel their weight,
As they drained my soul
To seal my fate!
I was being dragged down
Into utter despair,
Completely consumed by
Earth's many cares.
Gone was my joy, my peace,
My content.
As the thief came to steal
To destroy, his intent.
Lord "Help me"

Was my desperate plea,
"Restore my soul"
And to Him I did lean.
For the words once learned
Gleaned into sight,
"For my yoke is easy
And my burden is light."
So—over to Him,
I unloaded them all,
The weights I had carried,
I let them all fall!
He lifted me up,
As we communed there,
Our spirits made one,
As He and I shared.
Restored in His presence,
My soul free to soar.
His grace all sufficient,
My Saviour and Lord!

Edith Clattenburg
Used by permission by the author.

SURVIVAL GUIDE FOR CANCER

LEARN TO LIVE ONE DAY AT A TIME. Focus only on what needs to be done today—not tomorrow or the next day, just today. This takes practice. Our minds want to jump ahead. Strength comes in a one-day supply.

1. TAKE CARE OF YOURSELF. Eat healthily. My three major food groups are fruit, vegetables, and chocolate! Exercise as much as you are able. Going out for a walk can do wonders for your mental and physical health.

2. HAVE A GOOD SENSE OF HUMOUR. Be around people who make you laugh. Watch what you see on TV. Make sure you get in a few good belly laughs each day.

3. LEARN TO BE THANKFUL. What you are going through may not be the greatest, but there is always something to be thankful for. Try to look for at least five things each day. Doing so helps you to focus on the positive things.

4. DEVELOP A POSITIVE ATTITUDE. Read things that uplift you. Stay out of the medical books and off

the Internet for self-diagnosis. Leave that to the experts. Realize that you choose your attitude each day.

5. LIGHTEN UP! Let go of things that need to be let go of. Cancer puts things in perspective. Family, relationships, and health are important. Stuff isn't. If someone comes over for tea, use the good china, light the candles that have never been lit, and if something gets broken, oh well, that's just one less thing to pass on.

6. DO SOMETHING FOR OTHERS. There are always people who need your help. You may not be able to do much, but doing for someone else takes the focus off yourself.

7. TRUST GOD. A positive attitude can take you far. A positive faith can take you to infinity. Know that no matter the outcome, He is in control.

REFERENCES

Clairmont, Patsy. 1993. *Normal is Just a Setting on Your Dryer*. Colorado: Focus on the Family Publishing.

Clattenburg, Edith. "Burdens Lifted." Unpublished.

www.ingramcontent.com/pod-product-compliance
Lightning Source LLC
Chambersburg PA
CBHW050351290526
45785CB00006B/2731